I0490911

CONTENTS

GUIDE ON HOW TO GET PREGNANT EASILY: TIPS AND STRATEGIES

Introduction:

Getting pregnant is a significant milestone for many couples who are trying to start a family. However, it's important to note that achieving pregnancy isn't always as easy as it may seem for everyone. Factors such as age, health, and lifestyle choices can impact fertility levels and make it challenging for some couples to conceive. If you're planning to conceive and looking for ways to increase your chances of getting pregnant, this comprehensive guide will provide you with practical tips and strategies to help you on your journey towards parenthood.

Understanding the Menstrual Cycle: To increase your chances of getting pregnant, it's crucial to understand the menstrual cycle. The menstrual cycle is the regular hormonal cycle that occurs in women and prepares the body for pregnancy. It typically lasts for about 28 days, although it can vary for each individual. The menstrual cycle consists of several phases, including menstruation, follicular phase, ovulation, and luteal phase.

1. **Menstruation:** This is the phase when the uterine lining sheds, and bleeding occurs. It usually lasts for 3 to 7 days.

2. **Follicular Phase:** After menstruation, the follicular phase begins. During this phase, the follicle-stimulating hormone (FSH) is released, which stimulates the ovaries to produce mature eggs.

3. **Ovulation: Ovulation** is the most fertile phase of the menstrual cycle. It occurs when the mature egg is released from the ovary and travels towards the fallopian tube, where it can be fertilized by sperm. Ovulation usually occurs around the 14th day of a 28-day cycle, but it can vary for each woman.

4. **Luteal Phase:** After ovulation, the luteal phase begins. During this phase, the uterine lining thickens in preparation for a potential pregnancy. If the egg is not fertilized, the uterine lining will shed during the next menstrual cycle.

5. Knowing when you ovulate is crucial for timing intercourse and increasing your chances of getting pregnant. You can use various methods to track your ovulation, such as charting your basal body temperature, monitoring changes in cervical mucus, or using ovulation predictor kits.

MAINTAINING A HEALTHY LIFESTYLE:

Many couples dream of starting a family and having a child, but for some, the process of getting pregnant can be a bit more challenging than expected. While there is no magic formula for getting pregnant easily, there are several things you can do to increase your chances of conceiving. In this article, we will discuss some tips and techniques that can help you get pregnant more easily.

A healthy lifestyle plays a significant role in increasing fertility levels and improving the chances of getting pregnant. Here are some tips to maintain a healthy lifestyle:

1. **Eating a Balanced Diet**: A well-balanced diet that includes a variety of nutrients such as vitamins, minerals, protein, and healthy fats is crucial for reproductive health. Include plenty of fruits, vegetables, whole grains, lean proteins, and healthy fats in your diet. Avoid or limit foods that are high in sugar, unhealthy fats, and processed foods.

2. **Maintaining a Healthy Weight**: Both being overweight and underweight can impact fertility levels. Excess body weight can disrupt hormonal balance and affect ovulation, while being underweight can cause irregular periods or stop ovulation altogether. Maintain a healthy weight by eating a balanced diet and engaging in regular physical activity.

3. **Exercising Regularly**: Regular exercise can help

regulate hormones, improve overall health, and boost fertility levels. Aim for at least 30 minutes of moderate exercise most days of the week, such as walking, swimming, or yoga. Avoid excessive exercise, as it can disrupt hormonal balance and affect ovulation.

4. **Avoiding Smoking, Alcohol, and Drugs**: Smoking, alcohol, and recreational drugs can have detrimental effects on fertility. Smoking can damage the fallopian tubes and cervix, while excessive alcohol and drug use can disrupt hormonal balance and decrease sperm quality. It's best to quit smoking, limit alcohol intake, and avoid recreational

5. Understand your menstrual cycle: Understanding your menstrual cycle is one of the most important things you can do when trying to get pregnant. Your menstrual cycle is the series of changes your body goes through each month to prepare for a potential pregnancy. The cycle is measured from the first day of your period to the first day of your next period. Most women have a cycle that lasts between 28 and

32 days, but some women may have shorter or longer cycles. It is essential to track your menstrual cycle to know when you are ovulating. Ovulation is when an egg is released from the ovary and travels down the fallopian tube, where it can be fertilized by sperm. Ovulation typically occurs around day 14 of a 28-day cycle, but this can vary from woman to woman.

6. **Have regular sex**: To get pregnant, you need to have sex during your fertile window, which is the period of time when you are most likely to conceive. Your fertile window is the few days leading up to ovulation and the day of ovulation itself. Sperm can survive inside the female body for up to five days, so having sex in the days leading up to ovulation can increase your chances of conceiving.

It is recommended to have sex every two to three days throughout your menstrual cycle to ensure that sperm are always present in the reproductive tract. However, if you want to increase your chances of conceiving, you should focus on having sex during your fertile window.

To manage stress, try to incorporate stress-reducing techniques into your daily routine. This can include exercise, meditation, deep breathing, or yoga. Additionally, it is essential to prioritize self-care and take time for yourself to relax and unwind.

7. **Get enough sleep**:

Getting enough sleep is crucial for your overall health and

fertility. Lack of sleep can disrupt hormonal balance, which can affect ovulation and sperm production. Aim to get seven to eight hours of sleep each night and establish a consistent sleep schedule.

8. Consider using ovulation predictor kits:

Ovulation predictor kits can help you determine when you are ovulating and increase your chances of getting pregnant. These kits measure the levels of luteinizing hormone (LH) in your urine, which typically surge 24 to 48 hours before ovulation. When the kit detects the LH surge, it indicates that ovulation is likely to occur within the next day or two.

Using an ovulation predictor kit can help you time intercourse more accurately and increase your chances of conceiving. You can purchase these kits at most drug stores and online.

9. Consult with a healthcare provider:

If you have been trying to get pregnant for several months without success, it may be time to consult with a healthcare provider. They can help evaluate your fertility and recommend any necessary treatments.

Your healthcare provider may recommend fertility testing to determine if there are any underlying issues affecting your fertility. Treatment options may include medications, surgery, or assisted reproductive technologies, such as in vitro fertilization (IVF).

10. Have patience and stay positive:

Getting pregnant can take time, and it is important to have patience and stay positive throughout the process. It is normal for healthy couples to take up to a year or longer to conceive. Try to focus on the things you can control, such as maintaining a healthy lifestyle, and let go of things beyond your control.

MYTH VS. REALITY:

There are many myths and misconceptions about getting pregnant, and it can be hard to separate fact from fiction. Here are some common myths and the reality behind them:

Myth: You can get pregnant at any time of the month.

Reality: You can only get pregnant during a window of time known as the fertile window, which is typically five to six days before ovulation and the day of ovulation itself.

Myth: Having sex every day will increase your chances of getting pregnant.

Reality: Having sex every day can actually decrease sperm count and motility, which can reduce your chances of conceiving. Experts recommend having sex every other day during your fertile window.

Myth: Women can get pregnant at any age.

Reality: While women can get pregnant later in life, fertility declines as women age, and the risk of complications during pregnancy increases.

Myth: Stress can prevent you from getting pregnant.

Reality: While stress can affect hormonal balance and ovulation, occasional stress is unlikely to prevent you from getting pregnant.

However, chronic stress can have negative effects on overall health and fertility.

Myth: Certain sexual positions can increase your chances of getting pregnant.

Reality: There is no evidence to support the idea that certain sexual positions are more effective for getting pregnant. The most important factor is having regular sex during your fertile window.

Conclusion:

Getting pregnant can be an exciting and challenging journey, and there are many steps you can take to increase your chances of conceiving. By understanding your menstrual cycle, maintaining a healthy lifestyle, and seeking help when needed, you can improve your fertility and increase your chances of starting the family you have always wanted.

Remember that getting pregnant is a complex process influenced by many factors, and that it may take time and patience to achieve your goal. However, by staying positive, taking care of your body, and seeking support when needed, you can increase your chances of success and build the family you have always dreamed of.

WHEN TO SEEK HELP:

If you have been trying to conceive for six months to a year without success, it may be time to seek help from a fertility specialist. Women who are over 35 should consider seeking help after six months of trying, while women under 35 can wait up to a year.

A fertility specialist can help diagnose any underlying medical conditions that may be affecting your fertility, such as polycystic ovary syndrome (PCOS), endometriosis, or blocked fallopian tubes. They may also recommend fertility treatments such as ovulation induction, intrauterine insemination (IUI), or in vitro fertilization (IVF).

Remember that seeking help for fertility issues is nothing to be ashamed of. Infertility affects millions of couples worldwide, and there are many effective treatments available to help you conceive. By seeking help early, you can increase your chances of success and achieve your dream of starting a family.

Conclusion:

Getting pregnant can be a complex and challenging journey, but with the right tools and resources, you can increase your chances of success. By understanding your menstrual cycle, maintaining a healthy lifestyle, and seeking help when needed, you can improve your fertility and increase your chances of starting the family you have always wanted.

Remember that fertility is influenced by many factors, including age, genetics, and lifestyle, and that there is no guaranteed way to conceive. However, by staying positive, taking care of your body, and seeking support when needed, you can increase your chances of success and build the family you have always dreamed of.

ADDITIONAL TIPS:

1. Consider fertility-friendly lubricants:

Some lubricants can interfere with sperm motility and reduce your chances of getting pregnant. Consider using a fertility-friendly lubricant that is designed to mimic cervical mucus and help sperm move more easily. Examples of fertility-friendly lubricants include Pre-Seed and Conceive Plus.

2. Check your medications:

Some medications can affect fertility, so it is important to check with your healthcare provider about any prescription or over-the-counter medications you are taking. Some medications that can affect fertility include antidepressants, antipsychotics, chemotherapy drugs, and steroids.

3. Avoid exposure to toxins:

Exposure to toxins can affect both male and female fertility. Toxins can be found in the environment, in certain chemicals and pesticides, and in some household products. To reduce your exposure to toxins, avoid using harsh chemicals in your home, eat organic foods when possible, and limit your exposure to pollutants and chemicals in the air and water.

4. Keep track of your cervical mucus:

Cervical mucus is a fluid that is produced by the cervix throughout the menstrual cycle. As you approach ovulation, your cervical mucus will become thinner and more stretchy, which can help sperm move more easily through the cervix and into the fallopian tubes. By keeping track of your cervical mucus, you can help identify your most fertile days.

5. Consider acupuncture:

Acupuncture has been shown to improve fertility in some women. It may help improve blood flow to the uterus and ovaries, regulate hormonal balance, and reduce stress. If you are interested in acupuncture, be sure to find a licensed acupuncturist who specializes in fertility treatments.

6. Consider fertility supplements:

There are several supplements that may help improve fertility in both men and women. Examples of fertility supplements include folic acid, vitamin D, omega-3 fatty acids, and Coenzyme Q10 (CoQ10). However, it is important to talk to your healthcare provider before taking any supplements, as some may have side effects or interact with other medications.

In addition to seeking help from a fertility specialist, there are several other resources available to couples who are trying to conceive. These include:

1. Support groups: Joining a support group for couples who are trying to conceive can provide emotional support and valuable information about fertility treatments and strategies.

2. Fertility apps: There are several fertility apps

available that can help you track your menstrual cycle, predict ovulation, and monitor other important fertility indicators.

3. Fertility supplements: Some couples find that taking fertility supplements, such as folic acid, zinc, and vitamin D, can improve their chances of conceiving. However, it's important to talk to your doctor before taking any new supplements or medications.

4. Acupuncture: Some studies have suggested that acupuncture may improve fertility by reducing stress and improving blood flow to the reproductive organs.

5. Yoga and meditation: Practicing yoga and meditation can help reduce stress, improve hormone balance, and increase blood flow to the reproductive organs.

Ultimately, the key to getting pregnant easily is to understand your menstrual cycle, maintain a healthy lifestyle, and seek help when needed. By taking a proactive approach to your fertility and staying positive, you can increase your chances of success and achieve your dream of starting a family.

It's also important to remember that getting pregnant is not the only path to starting a family. Adoption and surrogacy are both viable options for couples who are struggling with infertility or other challenges.

Adoption is a wonderful way to build a family and provide a loving home to a child in need. There are many types of adoption available, including domestic adoption, international adoption, and foster care adoption. Each type of adoption has its own unique requirements and challenges, so it's important to do your research and choose the option that is best for you and your partner.

Surrogacy is another option for couples who are struggling with infertility or other challenges. In surrogacy, a woman carries a baby for another couple or individual who cannot carry a pregnancy themselves. Surrogacy can be a complex and expensive process, but it can also provide a wonderful opportunity for couples to start a family.

Whatever path you choose, remember that building a family is a journey that requires patience, perseverance, and a willingness to adapt to unexpected challenges. By staying positive, seeking help when needed, and remaining open to different options, you can achieve your dream of starting a family and experiencing the joys of parenthood.

It's also important to remember that the journey to starting a family can be emotionally challenging. Infertility, pregnancy loss, and other difficulties can take a toll on your mental health and your relationship with your partner. It's important to prioritize your emotional well-being and seek support when needed.

Here are some tips for coping with the emotional challenges of trying to conceive:

1. Seek support: Talk to friends, family members, or a therapist about your feelings and experiences. Join a support group for couples who are trying to conceive.

2. Practice self-care: Take time to do things you enjoy, such as reading, taking a bath, or going for a walk. Get plenty of rest, eat a healthy diet, and exercise regularly.

3. Communicate with your partner: Be open and honest with your partner about your feelings and concerns. Make time for each other and prioritize your relationship.

4. Manage stress: Try stress-reducing techniques such as meditation, yoga, or deep breathing exercises.

5. Set boundaries: If you're feeling overwhelmed by well-meaning family and friends who ask about your plans to have children, set boundaries and communicate your needs.

Remember that the emotional journey of starting a family can be just as important as the physical one. By taking care of your emotional well-being and seeking support when needed, you can navigate the ups and downs of trying to conceive and build a strong, healthy family.

Finally, it's important to remember that getting pregnant easily is not always possible. Infertility affects millions of couples worldwide, and it can be caused by a variety of factors including age, hormonal imbalances, genetics, and lifestyle choices. If you've been trying to conceive for a year or more without success, it may be time to seek help from a fertility specialist.

Fertility treatments such as in vitro fertilization (IVF), intrauterine insemination (IUI), and fertility drugs can help couples overcome infertility and increase their chances of conceiving. Your fertility specialist can help you determine the best treatment plan based on your individual needs and circumstances.

In some cases, couples may also consider using donor eggs, sperm, or embryos, or opting for a gestational carrier to carry the pregnancy. These options can be complex and expensive, but they can provide a wonderful opportunity for couples to start a family.

Remember that infertility is a medical condition, and seeking help from a fertility specialist is not a sign of weakness or failure. By taking a proactive approach to your fertility and seeking help when needed, you can increase your chances of success and achieve your dream of starting a family.

HERE'S AN EXAMPLE TO ILLUSTRATE THE POINT:

Sarah and John have been trying to conceive for several months without success. Sarah is 35 years old and has been tracking her menstrual cycle and taking prenatal vitamins, but they still haven't been able to get pregnant. They begin to feel discouraged and frustrated, and Sarah starts to worry that they will never be able to start a family.

At this point, Sarah and John decide to seek help from a fertility specialist. The specialist evaluates both partners and determines that Sarah has a hormonal imbalance that is affecting her fertility. They develop a treatment plan that includes fertility drugs to regulate her hormones and increase her chances of ovulating, as well as intrauterine insemination (IUI) to increase the chances of fertilization.

Despite their best efforts, Sarah and John still do not get pregnant after several rounds of IUI. At this point, they begin to consider other options, such as in vitro fertilization (IVF) or adoption. They take some time to discuss their options and weigh the pros and cons of each approach, and ultimately decide to pursue IVF.

After several months of preparing for IVF, Sarah undergoes the procedure and they are thrilled to learn that it is successful. Sarah gives birth to a healthy baby boy, and they feel grateful for the support of their fertility specialist and the many options available to them.

This example illustrates that getting pregnant easily is not always possible, and that infertility can be caused by a variety of factors. It also shows that seeking help from a fertility specialist and considering a range of options can increase the chances of starting a family.

Conclusion:

Getting pregnant can be a complex process, but by taking care of your health, understanding your menstrual cycle, and following the tips above, you can increase your chances of conceiving. Remember that fertility is influenced by many factors, including age, genetics, and lifestyle, and that there is no surefire way to guarantee pregnancy. However, by staying positive, taking care of your body, and seeking help when needed, you can improve your chances of getting pregnant and starting the family you have always wanted.

Remember, every person's body is different, and it may take some time to find what works best for you. If you have any concerns about your ability to conceive, speak to a healthcare professional.

ACKNOWLEDGEMENT

i will like to thank all who made this book possible to

ABOUT THE AUTHOR

Victor Ib

a passionate writer who loves making life easy

www.ingramcontent.com/pod-product-compliance
Lightning Source LLC
Chambersburg PA
CBHW071148220526
45467CB00015B/2118